American Ac...

DEDICATED TO THE

BLAST!

Babysitter **L**essons **A**nd
Safety **T**raining

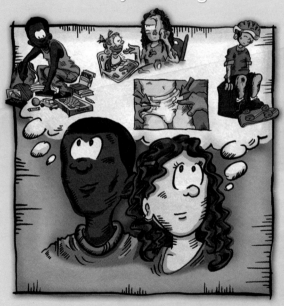

Second Edition

JONES & BARTLETT
LEARNING

World Headquarters
Jones & Bartlett Learning
5 Wall Street
Burlington, MA 01803
978-443-5000
info@jblearning.com
www.jblearning.com

American Academy of Pediatrics
DEDICATED TO THE HEALTH OF ALL CHILDREN®

Wendy Simon, MA, CAE, Director,
    Life Support Programs
Ellen Buerk, MD, MEd, FAAP, AAP
    Board Reviewer
David T. Tayloe, Jr, MD, FAAP, AAP
    Board Reviewer

American Academy of Pediatrics
141 Northwest Point Boulevard
Post Office Box 927
Elk Grove Village, IL 60009-0927
847-434-4798
www.aap.org

V.P., Production and Design:
    Anne Spencer
V.P., Manufacturing and Inventory Control:
    Therese Connell
Publisher, Public Safety: Kim Brophy
Publisher, Emergency Care:
    Lawrence D. Newell
Editor: Alton Thygerson, EdD, FAWM

Associate Editor: Janet Morris
Production Editor: Susan Schultz
Design: Nesbitt Graphics, Inc.
Typesetting: Spoke & Wheel
Illustrations: Dawn Griffin,
    Rolin Graphics
Printing and Binding: Transcontinental
    Printing

Jones & Bartlett Learning books and products are available through most bookstores and online booksellers. To contact Jones & Bartlett Learning directly, call 800-832-0034, fax 978-443-8000, or visit our website, www.jblearning.com.

Substantial discounts on bulk quantities of Jones & Bartlett Learning publications are available to corporations, professional associations, and other qualified organizations. For details and specific discount information, contact the special sales department at Jones & Bartlett Learning via the above contact information or send an e-mail to specialsales@jblearning.com.

Library of Congress Cataloging-in-Publication Data
BLAST : babysitter lessons and safety training / American Academy
of Pediatrics. — 2nd ed.
    p. cm.
    ISBN 13: 978-0-7637-3516-6 (pbk.) ISBN 10: 0-7637-3516-7 (pbk.)
    1. Babysitting—Juvenile literature. 2. Safety education—Juvenile literature.
    3. First aid in illness and injury—Juvenile literature.
    I. American Academy of Pediatrics.
  HQ769.5.B53 2006
  649'.1'0248--dc22
2006006490   6048
Printed in USA
15 14 13 12   11 10 9 8

Contents

Getting Started

As a babysitter, parent/guardian(s) trust you with their child's life. Your main responsibility is to care for a child's needs and keep the child safe. You can prepare yourself for these challenges by following the information in this manual and by completing the BLAST course.

When you are asked by a neighbor, friend, or relative to watch their child, you are being given a job that carries a big responsibility. Sitting is more than a way to earn money.

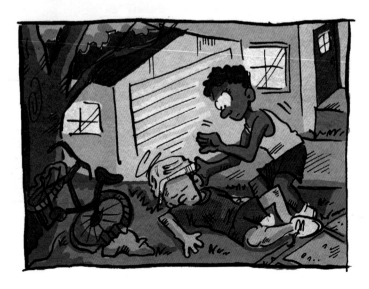

Are You Ready to Care for Children?

- Have your parent/guardian(s) help you decide if you are ready to take on this important job. With their help you should think about what you will and won't be able to handle as a babysitter. For example, you may decide to

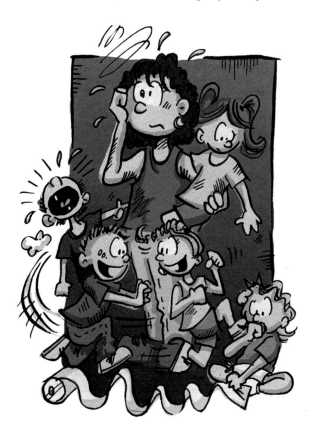

only watch children ages three and up or to only work on weekends. Are you mature enough to handle this job? A person must be at least 13 years old to take on the responsibility of watching young children and mature enough to handle common emergencies

- How many children can you handle at one time? A new sitter should start with one child or even start as a mother's helper. A more experienced sitter may handle several children of similar age. It takes a very experienced sitter to handle a mixed age group of children or more than three children at once. Watching too many children can challenge even a very experienced older teen sitter.

- Can you handle babies and young children? Younger teens should not sit for children less than six months old. Toddlers can also be challenging. Teens should only accept sitting for one child at a time if the child is three or younger.

- Have you been trained in how to care for small children? Have you received first aid and CPR training from a nationally recognized organization?

Discuss with parent/guardian(s) the proper time frame to watch children. A few hours for parent/guardian(s) to leave a young child in your care is acceptable, but all day or a very late night may not be. Contact your local child welfare agency, or check their website, to find out the time frame that you are legally able to watch a child in your state.

Sitter Qualities

Successful sitters have these
qualities. Are you?

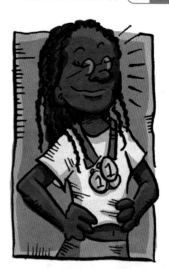

- Mature
- Trustworthy
- Patient
- Responsible
- Safety-conscious
- Fun-loving
- Punctual
- And do you like children

Be Prepared to Answer Questions

A responsible parent/guardian will interview sitters before
hiring them. They want to feel confident that you can do the
job. Expect to be asked these types of questions:

Experience

How much babysitting have you done? Have you cared for
other children the same age as theirs? Do you understand the
importance of constantly supervising the children?

Training

What training do you have in babysitting and first aid? Do
you know what to do in an emergency?

References

Can you provide names and phone numbers of families who
have hired you before? Are you responsible and trustworthy?

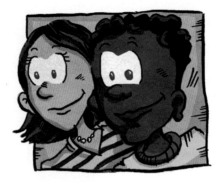

Availability

When can you sit? How late can you sit? What ages of children can you sit for?

Pay

Parent/guardian(s) may ask you what you charge. You should be prepared to tell them a rate per hour that is similar to what other sitters are being paid. You need to determine what sitters are getting paid per hour in your neighborhood. Ask friends who sit and parent/guardian(s) who hire sitters what a typical rate is. If the parent/guardian(s) do not ask what you charge, you may politely ask them what they will be paying per hour. It is OK for you to ask when they will pay you.

Be a Good Guest!

Remember that you are an invited guest in the house. The following rules are good to remember when sitting:

- Only eat food if you have been given permission to do so. If you are welcome to eat, clean up and wash any dishes when you are done.

- Avoid "exploring" another person's home, such as opening closets or drawers or looking through personal belongings.
- It would be best if friends did not visit you while sitting. This way your attention can always be on the child(ren).
- Avoid personal phone calls. The phone should be kept available for incoming calls from the child(ren)'s parent/guardian(s).

As They Grow: Ages and Stages

As children grow older they change. The table on the next page gives information about children as they move through different stages of growth. Remember that this chart is not the same for every child. Some can act differently even if they are the same age and in the same developmental stage.

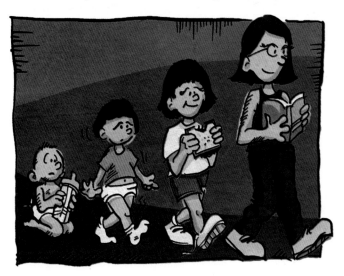

	Infant (0-1 years)	**Toddler** (1-3 years)
Communication	Responds to sound and touch. Uses eye contact. Begins to mimic sounds.	Begins to make sounds recognizable as early speech. Responds to tone of voice.
Care	Change diapers; bottle or spoon feed; burp; hold, and talk to infant.	Follow parent/guardian(s) guidelines. Help child use the toilet. Spoon feed, but help them feed themselves. Note foods to avoid for this age group on page 16. Help child wash hands and brush teeth.
Safety	Always place on back to sleep in the child's own crib. NEVER place an infant baby on a waterbed, beanbag, or anything that is soft enough to cover the face and block air to the nose and mouth. No bedding or soft toys should be placed in the crib.	Gets into everything, very curious. Keep child away from choking hazards. Monitor their eating. Limit play space.
Play	Plays alone with rattles, stuffed animals, and mobiles. Uses eye contact. Reaches for things.	Plays separately from others. May watch others play, but usually won't share or interact. Enjoys being read to and simple games.
Misbehavior	Disciplining not needed. Follow parent/ guardian(s) guidelines.	Use time-out or distraction. Follow parent/ guardian(s) guidelines.

Preschool **(3-5 years)**	**School Age** **(5-8 years)**
A 3–5 year old has a very large vocabulary. Can say anything he or she wants and often makes 5 word sentences.	Can talk with you, but vocabulary probably smaller than yours.
Follow parent/guardian(s) guidelines. Let them eat with their hands. Don't force child to eat. Help child use the toilet if needed. Help child wash hands and brush teeth.	Should be able to use the toilet alone. Remind them to wash hands afterwards and before meals. May want to help you or may have chores to do.
Children are very mobile; limit play area. Monitor their playing.	Know where they are at all times. DO NOT let them do anything that makes you uncomfortable. Children need boundaries.
Enjoys active physical games with interaction (tag, hide-and-seek). Enjoys being read to.	Enjoys organized games.
Give yes or no choices. Follow parent/guardian(s) guidelines.	Can reason with child. Follow parent/guardian(s) guidelines.

Before Saying "Yes" to a Job

Part of taking a sitting job seriously is protecting yourself as well as the children for whom you will be caring. Know the people you are sitting for before you take the job. Check references if this will be the first time working for this person. Get the parent/guardian's name, address, and phone number. Your parent(s) may want to meet the people you are sitting for if they are not already acquainted.

Get specific instructions about the number and ages of the children, bed times, foods, medicines, and other information about personal habits as well as what is expected of you. Parent/guardian(s) typically feel confident with a sitter who asks questions and who is concerned with the care of the children. Discuss the information with your parent/guardian(s) before accepting the job. Use the Sitter's Checklist (pages 32, 33).

You may find enough jobs simply by letting friends and neighbors know that you are available to babysit. It is not a good idea to post flyers on supermarket bulletin boards or on the street or to place a classified ad in newspapers or to have a website. You may receive some unwelcome responses, and it may not be safe. While most people are nice, do not make it easy for a stranger to find out your age, where you live, or your email address.

Accept jobs only from people you already know or from those that are recommended to you. Accepting jobs from strangers is not as safe as sitting for a neighbor or a neighbor's friend. If you do not know the person calling, ask who recommended you, and tell the caller that you will call him/her back. If you do not know the people you plan to sit for, bring a trusted adult (parent/guardian(s), adult friend, etc.) along for the interview. The adult is there for support and safety. You should answer any questions and be prepared to ask questions. If you have any doubt or feel uneasy or fearful about the person or situation, refuse the job. Other jobs will become available.

A Few Important Points

- Let your parent/guardian(s) know where and when you are sitting.
- Always leave information telling them:
  - Name, address, and phone number of the people for whom you are sitting.
  - Time you will be brought home or need your parent/guardian or other family member to pick you up from the sitting job.

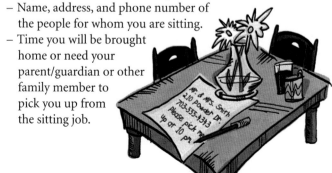

- Arrange your own transportation to get to the location and to return home. If a family member is not picking you up, call home to let someone know that you are on your way. Never accept rides from people who have been drinking alcohol.
- Be sure you have an escort home. This should be either a parent/guardian or family member. Never go home alone from a night job.
- Learn how to use any electronic security system if the home has one.
- Let the parent/guardian(s) you are sitting for know if you have a curfew. Ask them to call if they are running late.
- Call the parent/guardian(s) about a problem such as:
  - If a child has been crying for longer than 20 minutes and you can't figure out what's wrong;
  - If a child develops a fever, vomits, or is injured (more than a superficial scrape);
  - Anytime a situation develops that you feel you can't handle without help.

You should also call your own parent/guardian(s) for advice and assistance if something arises.

When a Stranger Calls

- Always keep the doors locked when caring for a child.
- Never allow strangers into the house unless the family members specifically informed you that a person would be coming over, such as a neighbor to pick up some items.

- Keep the door closed unless you know the person. Call the police if someone insists on coming in and you do not recognize the person, or if you suspect a prowler. If you must open the door to talk, keep any chain lock fastened until you are sure that it is safe.
- If someone calls, there is no reason to tell a caller that you are a sitter for the children. If you do, this implies that you are alone in the house. If asked, respond by saying that you are visiting, and the child(ren)'s parent/guardian(s) cannot come to the phone. Ask to take a message. Tell the caller that the person will return the call shortly.
- Stay inside with the doors locked if you hear suspicious noises or activities outside. Attempting to investigate could be dangerous. Stay inside. Turn on outside lights, and call the police if you suspect a prowler. Be sure that all doors and windows are locked.

House Rules and Routines

Parent/guardian(s) should provide you with each of these items before they leave their children in your care:

- Acceptable television programs, computer games, and movies;
- Food and eating times;
- Guidelines for outside play, such as instructions about protective gear for bikes, skateboards, scooters, inline skates, and proper clothing, what to do and where to do it;

- Information on allergies or illness
- Guidelines for having child(ren)'s friends visit;
- Bedtime routine;
- Special considerations;
- Parent/guardian(s)' discipline practices—what should you do if a child breaks a rule (time out, to bed early, etc.);
- Rooms off-limits to the children;
- Note: If the child has an allergy that may require the use of an epi pen, the parents should let you know where the pen is kept and give guidance for its use.

Safety Rules

- Never leave children unattended with small objects. Any food given to children under age four should be cut into tiny pieces (about the size of a child's fingertip). Any toys that can fit inside a toilet paper tube may be too small, and the child could choke on the object if

Choking Hazards

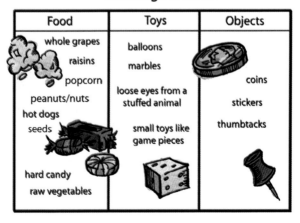

Food	Toys	Objects
whole grapes	balloons	coins
raisins	marbles	stickers
popcorn	loose eyes from a stuffed animal	thumbtacks
peanuts/nuts		
hot dogs	small toys like game pieces	
seeds		
hard candy		
raw vegetables		

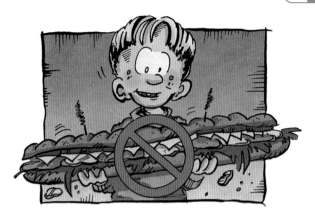

swallowed. Any objects left on the floor, like a coin, can quickly become an object that could choke a child who places it in his or her mouth.

- While holding a baby or young child, you should not eat or drink.
- Medicine should only be given with the parent/ guardian's permission. Follow instructions carefully.
- Be alert when a child is near water. Only sponge baths should be given. A child should never be left alone in a bathtub. Children can drown in only a few inches of water if they are not watched carefully. Also, pools and spas should not be accessible.
- Always dress children properly for outdoor play activities.
- Keep children away from electrical outlets, stairs, and stoves.
- Check a sleeping child often.
- Supervise children at all times, especially in the kitchen and bathroom.

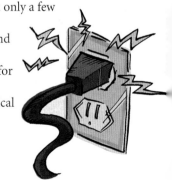

Safe House

Bedroom 2 – for infant
- Changing table with strap to secure infant
- Keep changing table away from windows
- Electrical outlets covered

Kitchen
- Pot handles turned in
- Back burners used
- Hot fluids/food kept out of reach
- Appliances and electrical cords kept out of reach
- Electrical outlets covered
- Cabinets & oven with childproof locks
- Chairs kept away from sink and stove
- Locking trashcan
- Proper highchair for feeding
- Knives/sharp objects put away or protected

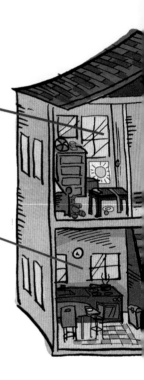

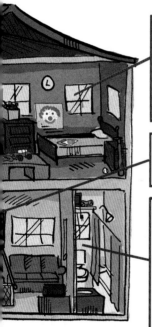

Bedroom 1 – for young child
- Windows/screens secured
- No chairs in front of windows
- Electrical outlets covered
- Small toys or games with small pieces stored away

Stairs
- Locking gates at top and bottom of stairs

Bathroom
- Non-skid surfaces
- Locking trashcan
- Cabinets with childproof locks
- Water temperatures set to avoid burning
- Appliances and electrical cords kept out of reach
- Toilet seat down

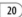

Fire

- Plan ahead. Know how to get yourself and the children out of the house in case of fire. Walk through the house with the parent/guardian(s) to ensure all doors and windows are locked and to locate how to leave the house in case of a fire. You should ask the parent/guardian(s) about a pre-arranged safe meeting place.

In Case of Fire or if the Smoke Alarm Goes Off...

- Remain calm and think about the exit routes you located previously.
- Sound the alarm—yell "FIRE!" as loud as possible.
- Test doors before you open them. Touch the door with the back of your hand—at the knob and around the frame. If there is a fire on the other side, it will feel warm on the knob and around the cracks. If the door is warm, try another escape route.
- If possible, close the door to the area where the fire is. Smoke kills and shutting doors stops it from advancing.
- Leave the fire alone. Attempt to save lives—yours and the child(ren)'s.
- Get everyone out of the house immediately, and do not go back in for any reason. Children may try to return to the house to "save" a pet or favorite toy or blanket. Many people are killed returning to a burning building.
- Keep all the children together. Go to a known neighbor's house.
- Call, or have the neighbor call, the emergency telephone number (usually 9-1-1). Then, call the parent/guardian(s).

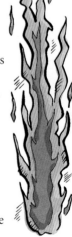

Diapering

1. Get Ready. Have everything you need within reach. Never leave a baby unattended, even for a second. Wash your hands.

2. Cover the changing surface (crib, floor, or changing table) with a towel or changing cloth. If using a changing table, use the safety restraint.

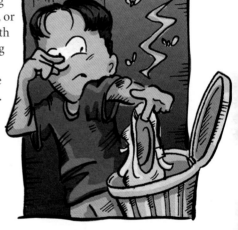

3. Remove the dirty diaper. As you remove the diaper, notice how it was secured. Hold the baby's ankles and carefully lift the hips.

4. Wipe in the correct direction. Using a warm washcloth or baby wipes, gently wipe the baby clean from the front to the back. Wiping from back to front, especially on girls, could spread germs that can cause an infection. Wipe the creases in the thighs and buttocks. Keep a clean diaper over a baby boy's penis since he could spray you, the walls, or anything else in range.

5. Dry the baby with a clean washcloth, and apply diaper ointment if needed.
6. Put on a clean diaper. Gently lift the legs and feet and slide the diaper under the baby. Bring the bottom half of the diaper up through the baby's legs. A boy's penis should be placed downward before fastening the diaper to prevent leaks above the waistline.
7. Fasten the diaper. Bring the adhesive strips of the disposable diaper around and fasten snugly. Avoid sticking the tape onto the baby's skin.
8. Get rid of the diaper. If a disposable diaper, empty any bowel movements in the toilet and properly dispose of diaper.
9. Change any wet or dirty baby clothes.
10. Wash your hands thoroughly after changing a baby's diaper to avoid getting sick.

Be prepared to help toddlers who have recently been "potty trained." They may still need help with undressing, wiping, and washing hands.

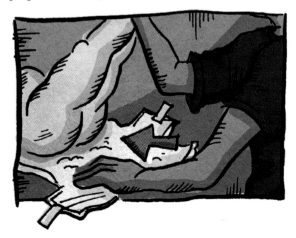

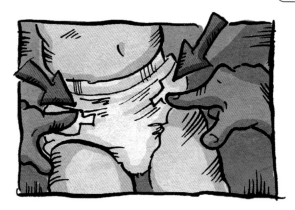

Bottle Feeding

- Wash your hands before and after feeding the baby. No health reason exists for feeding a baby warmed milk, but most babies prefer it. You can warm a bottle in a pan of hot—not boiling—water or by running it under the hot water tap, or use a commercial bottle warmer if available. A microwave should not be used to heat a milk bottle since it can cause burns.

- Test the milk's temperature by sprinkling a few drops of it on the inside of your wrist before giving it to the baby. If it is too hot on your wrist, it is too hot for the baby. Let it cool and retest before giving it to the baby.

- If you offer a bottle and the baby doesn't immediately start sucking, try stroking his or her cheek with your finger. When the mouth opens, insert the nipple completely and make sure it's on top of the tongue, not under it. If he or she isn't awake or alert enough to eat, you can try rousing the baby by sitting him or her up or taking off a layer of clothing to make the baby cooler.

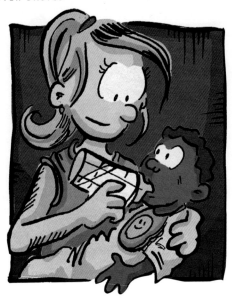

- The best position for feeding a baby is sitting in an armchair or rocking chair with your elbows and arms supported. If you feel any strain, put pillows under your arms or under the baby until you find a comfortable feeding position. Hold the baby semi-upright in your lap, and cradle his or her head in the crook of your arm. (Make sure the head is higher than the torso. Otherwise fluid can collect in the Eustachian tubes and affect the middle ear, causing an ear infection.) Propping the bottle in the baby's mouth can cause tooth decay or choking. Always stay with the baby, and keep bottles out of the baby's crib. Hold the bottle so the milk fills the neck of the bottle and covers the nipple. This will prevent the baby from swallowing air as he or she sucks.

Burping a Baby

Even when the flow of liquid is perfect, if babies swallow some air they can become fussy or spit up if they are not burped often. Try burping after every two to three ounces (about one-third) of a bottle. One sign that an air bubble in the stomach may bother him or her is that he or she stops eating before you'd expect him or her to be full. Try these three easy burping methods:

- Hold the baby upright against your shoulder and chest and support the back. Rub, pat, or massage his or her back with your other hand.
- Sit the baby on one side of your lap, support his or her chest with your opposite hand, lean the baby slightly forward, and with your other hand, rub or pat his/her back.
- Lay the baby face down across your lap—stomach on one leg and the head on the other leg. Support his or her head so it is higher than the chest. Gently rub or pat his or her back

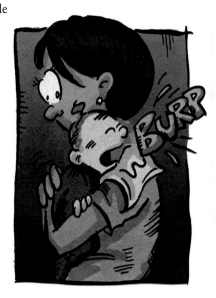

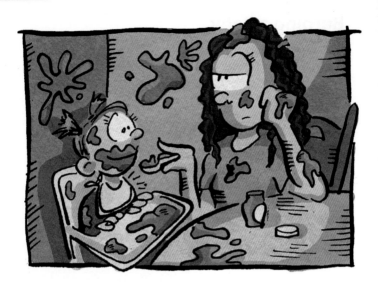

Spoon Feeding Baby/Toddler

1. Wash your hands before and after feeding the child.
2. Get the food ready before putting the child into the chair or seat. Put the baby food in a dish and put a bib under chin and on chest.
3. Secure the child in the seat with a safety belt if available and lock the tray in place.
4. Test to see that the food's temperature is OK.
5. Use a small spoon and put about a quarter teaspoonful on its tip. If a child doesn't want to eat, that is OK.
6. When finished, wash the child's hands and face, and wipe up any spilled food.

Crying

You can get frustrated when a baby cries, especially if it goes on without stopping. The longer the baby cries, the more difficult the crying will be to stop. Babies cry for many reasons: full diaper, empty bottle, or air in the stomach (keep the baby upright during feeding to reduce air intake). Changing the physical surroundings may help stop the crying. Try one or more of the following methods to get the baby to stop crying:

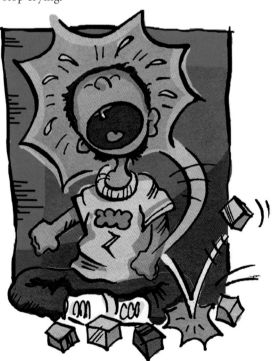

1. Go for a walk with the baby in a carrier, a sling, or your arms.
2. Rock the baby in your arms, a cradle, a baby swing, or a carriage.
3. Talk to the baby.
4. Cuddle the baby.
5. Sing a song to the baby.
6. Massage the baby's back, arms, or legs.
7. Use a pacifier.
8. Place the baby in the crib or playpen, walk away, and take a few minutes to calm down.

Ask the parents/guardians at what point they would like to be called if attempts to calm the child do not work. You can suggest calling them after 20 to 30 minutes of continuous crying.

Shaken Baby Syndrome

A crying baby can frustrate a caregiver. Never react to crying by shaking a baby. This can damage the brain. Mild shaking over time can cause learning disabilities and attention deficit disorder. Severe shaking, even once, can cause paralysis, blindness, hearing loss, and death.

Preparing for Bed

Bedtime can sometimes create anxiety for young children. Here are some tips for making bedtime fun for each age group:

Infants

- Ask the parent/guardian about the usual "bedtime routine" for the baby.

- Gently rub the baby on the back before putting him/her in the crib.
- Lay the baby on his or her back, and take all stuffed toys out of the crib.
- Play soft music.
- Once the baby is calm, try sitting quietly in the room.
- If the baby cries a lot, help him or her to relax and settle down to sleep.
- Make sure the baby is asleep and turn on the baby monitor and night light before you leave the room.

Toddlers

- Ask the parent/guardian the best methods to get the child to sleep.
- Encourage quiet time as bedtime approaches.
- Make reading or story-telling a fun part of bedtime.
- Stay in the room until the child is asleep.
- Turn on a nightlight(s) if appropriate.
- Place the door to the room according to the parent/guardian(s) and child's request (leave the door open slightly).

Preschoolers

- Ask the parent/guardian what the child likes to do to get ready for sleep.
- Keep activities calm before naptime or going to bed.
- Read a book together.
- Relax and play imagination games to help the preschooler close his or her eyes.

School-Age Children

- Ask the parent/guardian what time the child should be in bed, and what time he or she should be asleep.

- Older children may want to read, or have you read to them, before they go to sleep.
- Play soothing music.
- Play imagination games.
- Assure children that their parent/guardian(s) will be home when they wake up.

Behavior Problems

Children may misbehave for a sitter, even more than for a parent/guardian. Causes for misbehavior include:

- Tired
- Ill
- Hungry or thirsty
- Bored
- Frustrated
- Too much excitement
- Scared
- Needs attention

Discipline

Getting children to behave can sometimes be a challenge. See the tips in the Sitter's Checklist to help you deal with discipline issues.

Sitter's Checklist

Give the following checklist to the parent/guardian(s) ahead of time or let the parent/guardian(s) know that you will arrive early for them to fill it out.

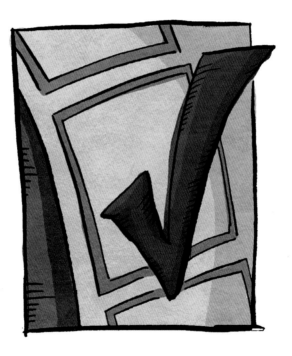

Sitter's Checklist ✔

Parent/guardian(s) first & last names	
House address	
Nearest cross streets/ intersection	
House phone number	
Where are the telephones located?	
Where parent/guardian(s) will be?	
When will parent/guardian(s) return?	
Phone number to contact parent/guardian(s)	
Neighbors' names and phone numbers if parent/guardian(s) cannot be reached	First neighbor: Second neighbor:
Emergency phone number	9-1-1 – if not, it is:
Poison Control Center phone	1-800-222-1222
Name and phone number of doctor	
Where are first aid supplies?	
Where is a flashlight?	
How do I lock the door, windows, and security system?	
Where are the best routes out of the house in case of a fire?	
Nightlight on? Yes or No	
Pets' name(s) and care	
Child #1 name Age Nap and/or bed times	

Special instructions • food allergies • medical condition(s) • names of medication(s) and dosages • how to help the child in the bathroom • what, how much, and when to feed • discipline	
Child #2 name Age Nap and/or bed times Special instructions • food allergies • medical condition(s) • names of medication(s) and dosages • how to help the child in the bathroom • what, how much, and when to feed • discipline	
Child #3 name Age Nap and/or bed times Special instructions • food allergies • medical condition(s) • names of medication(s) and dosages • how to help the child in the bathroom • what, how much, and when to feed • discipline	
Routines to follow	
Rules and restrictions	
Other special instructions	

First Aid

What to Do for an Injured or Sick Child

What is not an Emergency?

Some problems need your quick help but are not emergencies. Examples include: small cuts, slight fevers, diarrhea or stomachaches, earaches, minor bruises, nosebleeds, rashes, or sprained ankles. You can handle most of these problems yourself. If you are not sure about what to do for a problem that is not an emergency, call the parent/guardian(s) or the child's doctor.

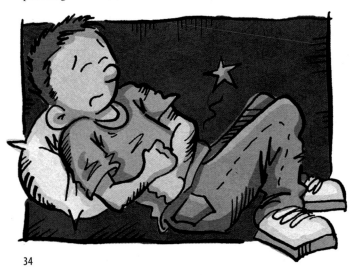

What is an Emergency?

An emergency is when you believe a severe injury or illness is threatening a child's health or may cause permanent harm. In these cases, a child needs emergency medical treatment right away. Examples of emergencies include:

- Unresponsiveness (the child cannot wake up or respond to you)
- Seizures or convulsions (bad shaking that will not stop)
- Choking on food, drink, or an object
- Falls from high places
- Severe burns
- Trouble breathing
- Eating or drinking something poisonous
- Heavy bleeding that will not stop
- Cannot move arms or legs

Calling 9-1-1 for Help

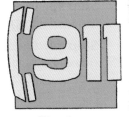

Any time you think a child is in danger, immediately call the emergency telephone number (usually 9-1-1 in most cities and towns) for help. Be ready to tell the 9-1-1 dispatcher the following:

- Your name and the phone number you are calling from
- What happened, who it happened to
- Exact address of the emergency and the closest major cross streets/intersection

Wait for the dispatcher to hang up. The dispatcher may keep you on the line and be able to tell you how to care for the child until the ambulance arrives.

After you have called your local EMS, contact the child's parent(s) or legal guardian(s).

CPR: Child (ages 1–8 years)

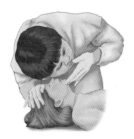 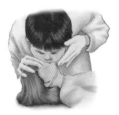

Step #1. Check for responsiveness by shouting, "Are you OK?" and tapping the child.

Step #2. Have someone call 9-1-1. If alone, provide about 2 minutes of care if you are sure of what to do. Otherwise, call 9-1-1 and follow the dispatcher's instructions.

Step #3. Open airway by tilting the head back with one hand and lifting the chin up with the other hand.

Step #4. Check breathing by looking at the chest to see if it rises and falls, and listen and feel for air at the mouth.

If...	Then...
breathing	roll child onto side.
not breathing	pinch nose and give 2 breaths making the chest rise with each breath.
breath does not make the chest rise	retilt the head and try breaths again. If chest does not rise, begin CPR (see step #5). When opening airway to give a breath, look for an object in the throat and if seen, remove it.
2 breaths make chest rise	continue to step #5.

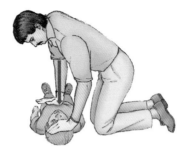

Step #5. Give CPR.

- Place heel of 1 or 2 hands on the center of the chest. Do not press near the bottom tip of the breastbone.
- If using one hand for compressions, use your other hand to keep head tilted.
- Press down quickly on the chest 1 to 1 ½ inches deep and release 30 times (rate of 100 compressions per minute—count 1, 2, 3, 4, 5).
- Give 2 slow breaths after every 30 compressions.

After about 2 minutes, recheck breathing. If alone or if no one has called yet, call 9-1-1. If there are no signs of breathing, continue CPR.

Choking: Child (ages 1–8 years)

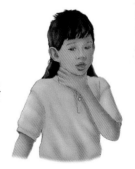

Step #1. Ask child if he/she is choking. Being unable to talk or cough are signs of choking.

Step #2. Give abdominal thrusts.

- Stand or kneel behind the child, and wrap your arms around the child.

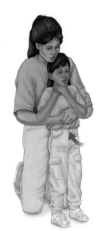

- Place the thumb side of your fist against the child's abdomen just above the navel.
- Grab the fist with your other hand and press into the child's stomach with quick upward thrusts until the object is removed or the child becomes unresponsive.
- If child becomes unresponsive, call 9-1-1 for help, and begin CPR (before giving a breath, look for an object in the throat and if seen, remove it).

CPR: Infant (less than 1 year old)

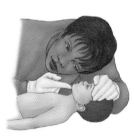

Step #1. Check for responsiveness by shouting, "Are you OK?" and gently tapping the baby.

Step #2. Have someone call 9-1-1. If alone, provide about 2 minutes of care if you are sure of what to do. Otherwise, call 9-1-1 and follow the dispatcher's instructions.

Step #3. Open airway by gently tilting the head back slightly with one hand and lifting the chin up with the other hand.

Step #4. Check breathing by looking at the chest to see if it rises and falls and listen and feel for air at the mouth.

If...	Then...
breathing	roll baby onto side.
not breathing	give 2 breaths to make chest rise. Cover the mouth and nose with your mouth.
breath does not make the chest rise	retilt the head and try breaths again. If chest does not rise, begin CPR (see step #5). When opening airway to give a breath, look for an object in the throat and if seen, remove it.
2 breaths make chest rise	continue to step #5.

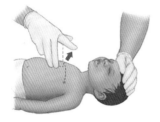 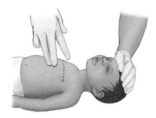

Step #5 Give CPR.

- Place 2 fingers of 1 hand on the center of the infant's breastbone about 1 finger's width below the imaginary line drawn between the infant's nipples. Avoid bottom of breast bone.
- Use your other hand to keep head tilted.
- Press down quickly on the chest ½ to 1 inch deep and release 30 times (rate of at least 100 compressions per minute—count 1, 2, 3, 4, 5).
- Give 2 breaths after every 30 compressions.

After about 2 minutes, recheck breathing. Call 9-1-1 if no one has already done so. If no signs of breathing, continue CPR.

Choking: Infant (less than 1 year old)

If infant is responsive but cannot cry, breathe, or cough:

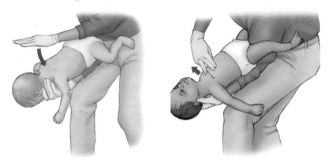

Step #1. Hold infant's head and neck with 1 hand by supporting infant's jaw between your thumb and fingers.

Step #2. Place infant facedown over your forearm with head lower than his or her chest. Brace your forearm and infant against your leg.

Step #3. Give 5 back blows between the infant's shoulder blades with the heel of your free hand.

Step #4. Give 5 chest thrusts. Turn infant onto his or her back while supporting head. Use 2 fingers over the breastbone as you would in giving CPR but at a slower rate. Continue back blows and chest thrusts until object is removed or child becomes unresponsive.

Step #5. If infant becomes unresponsive, call 9-1-1 for help, and begin CPR. Before giving a breath, look for an object in the throat and if seen, remove it.

Bleeding and Shock

1. Using a sterile dressing or clean, dry cloth, press on the wound to stop bleeding. Wear disposable medical exam gloves from a first aid kit if available.

2. If bleeding is from an arm or leg, raise the arm or leg while still pressing on the wound, unless the arm or leg is broken.

3. Shallow wounds can be washed with clean, running water. Apply a bandage and follow up with the parent(s) or legal guardian(s). For a deep wound, do not try to clean the wound or apply antibiotic ointment. A deep wound requires cleaning by a medically trained person. Call parent/guardian(s) and 9-1-1.

When someone suffers a serious injury and loses a lot of blood, shock can occur. The signs of shock include anxiousness, dizziness, fast heartbeat and fast breathing, and cool, moist, pale skin. Care for shock by lying the victim on his/her back, raising the legs 8"–12", keeping the victim warm, and calling 9-1-1.

Bone, Joint, and Muscle Injuries

The child may be unable to move or use the injured body part after falling or being hit. The body part may also be deformed, tender when touched, painful, and/or swollen.

Use RICE for care:

R = Rest: Keep the body part in place and out of use.

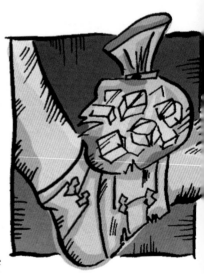

I = Ice: Cover the injury with a wet cloth and apply ice or a cold pack for periods of 20 minutes every 2 hours.

C = Compression: When not applying an ice bag, wrap an elastic bandage around the body part if one is available.

E = Elevation: Raise the injured body part above the heart level. by placing the injured limb on several pillows.

- Call parent/guardian(s) or neighbor.

If you suspect a broken bone or injured joint:

- Keep the body part in place.
- Stabilize the part by holding it still.
- Call 9-1-1 and parent/guardian(s) or neighbor.

Breathing Difficulty

For asthma:

If a child has asthma and a doctor-prescribed hand-held inhaler, ask a parent/guardian to demonstrate its use before leaving the child in your care.

1. Keep the child upright.
2. If the child has a doctor-prescribed hand-held inhaler, give it to the child. He or she will know how to use it.
3. Give the child water to drink if they can swallow.
4. Call parent/ guardian(s).

For hyperventilation (breathing too fast):

1. Reassure and calm the child.
2. Encourage the child to take long, slow breaths and to hold each breath for about 3 to 5 seconds before slowly exhaling.

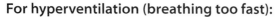

Burns

1. Apply cool water or cool, wet cloths until the pain stops.
2. After the pain has stopped:

If...	Then...
minor burns (red skin), such as from a sunburn	• apply a clean dry gauze pad over the the burned area • do not apply burn ointments or petroleum jelly to the burn • do not break any blisters
severe burns (blisters, discolored skin)	• call 9-1-1 and parent/ guardian(s) or neighbor.

Chemical burn:

1. Flush with running water for about 15 minutes (until an ambulance arrives).
2. Call 9-1-1 and parent/guardian(s) or neighbor.

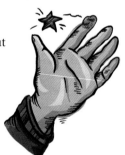

Diabetic Emergencies

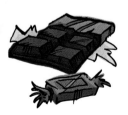

The parent/guardian(s) should tell you if their child is diabetic. Before leaving, parent/guardian(s) should also tell you how to recognize and handle a diabetic emergency. Suspect an emergency if the child starts to mumble, fumble, stumble and is not alert.

1. If the child is old enough, ask the child to check his or her blood sugar, and then call the parents with the results.
2. If the child cannot check blood sugar, but can swallow, give some food or drink containing sugar. Examples: table sugar, soda, or fruit juice.
3. If not better in 10-15 minutes, give the child more sugar and call parent/guardian(s). If unresponsive, call 9-1-1.

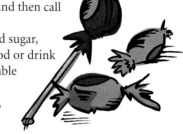

Diarrhea

Diarrhea is frequent, watery, mushy stool, and can have several causes. Have the child drink lots of fluids.

1. Most children should continue eating a normal diet including formula or milk while they have mild diarrhea.
2. Some children are not able to tolerate cow's milk when they have diarrhea and it may be temporarily removed from the diet.
3. If child wears diapers, change them immediately and clean the child after each diarrhea episode. Apply petroleum jelly. Wash your hands after every diaper change or toilet assistance.

Dog Bite

Take caution around family
pets. Follow these rules to
keep yourself and the
children safe:

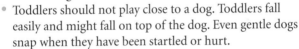

- Children should not be left
  alone in a room with a dog.
- Keep children away from
  eating or sleeping dogs.
- Children should not tease
  or hurt dogs.
- Toddlers should not play close to a dog. Toddlers fall
  easily and might fall on top of the dog. Even gentle dogs
  snap when they have been startled or hurt.
- If a dog scares you, you can refuse to sit for the family.

In case of dog bite:

1. Place a sterile dressing or clean, dry cloth over the bite site.
2. Press on the wound to stop bleeding.
3. After bleeding has stopped, wash the bite wound with soap
   and water.
4. Cover the bite wound with a sterile dressing or clean cloth.
5. Call parent/guardian(s) or neighbor.
6. If the animal is unknown, get a good description of it.
7. If the animal is a family pet, isolate it.

Electrocution

If...	Then...
child is still touching wire, appliances, etc.,	turn off the power source before you touch the child so you do not become electrocuted.
the child is unresponsive	use the methods described in the Rescue Breathing and CPR section. Call 9-1-1.
the child is responsive	call parent/guardian(s).

Eye Injuries

If...	Then...
an object is stuck in the child's eye	call 9-1-1. Leave the object where it is. Call the parent/guardian(s) or neighbor. Attempt to cover the injured eye with an eye shield or paper cup.
chemical is in child's eye	flush the eye with lukewarm water for 15 to 20 minutes. Call the parent/guardian(s) or neighbor.
a loose object (eyelash, dust, dirt, etc.) is in the child's eye	gently grasp the upper lid and pull it out and down over the lower eyelid. Tears that occur when you pull the upper lid over the lower lid may help dislodge the object.

Fever

Fever—a high body temperature (over 98.6° F)—is developed by the body to fight an infection. Fever helps fight infection. A fever in a child under three months of age needs medical attention. Fever can cause a seizure that can be frightening but does not usually result in serious problems.

If the child is younger than 3 years of age, taking his or her temperature with a rectal digital thermometer provides the best reading. Taking an oral temperature is not recommended for young children because they cannot hold the thermometer under the tongue with the mouth closed. Ear thermometers are also acceptable.

To help reduce fever:

1. Give sips of water, crushed ice, or electrolyte solutions.
2. Call the parent/guardian(s) before giving acetaminophen when the fever is above 101°F. *Aspirin should not be given to a child.*
3. Dress the child in light clothing, but do not allow the child to shiver. Shivering increases the body temperature.
4. Bathing with lukewarm water helps bring down fever. Cold water or rubbing alcohol should not be used to bathe a child.
5. For a high fever (105°F or higher), which can be a sign that the child has a potentially serious problem, call the parent/guardian(s) or neighbor.

Head Injuries

If...	Then...
bleeding from scalp	apply gentle pressure to control any bleeding. Call parent/guardian(s) or neighbor. For shallow scalp wound, flush with water from a faucet. Put a clean bandage on the wound once the bleeding has stopped.
swelling appears and is painful	apply ice pack for 15 to 20 minutes.
child does not move	see CPR section. If breathing, place child on left side to keep airway open, to drain fluids, and to handle possible vomiting.

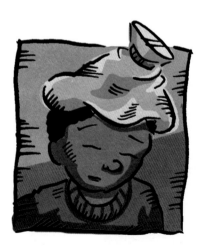

Insect Stings

*If the child has a known allergy to insect
stings and has a doctor-prescribed EpiPen, a
parent/guardian should let you know
where the pen is kept and give guidance for
its use before leaving the child in your care.*

1. Wash stung area with soap and water.
   For a honeybee, look for a stinger in the
   skin and if found, scrape or brush it out with a
   long fingernail or similar object.
2. Apply ice bag for 15 to 20 minutes.
3. Observe for breathing difficulty and swollen face and if
   found, call parent/guardian(s) or neighbor. For very
   difficult breathing, call 9-1-1. If the child is known to be
   allergic to insect stings and has a doctor-prescribed
   epinephrine kit, use it.

Nosebleed

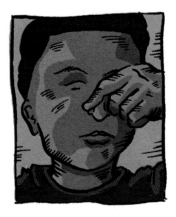

1. Keep child in sitting
   position leaning slightly
   forward. Remind child to
   breathe through the mouth.
2. Pinch both nostrils with
   steady pressure for ten
   minutes. If able, the child
   can do the pinching.
3. If bleeding continues for
   more than 30 minutes, call
   parent/guardian(s)
   or neighbor.

Poisoning

Poisoning is one of the most common childhood injuries. Children between the ages of eight months and six years old are the most likely to be poisoned. Poisons can look like things that are good to eat and drink. They can come in many colors and forms, including solids, liquids, sprays, or gases. Young children are curious. They like to put things in their mouths, especially if they look colorful or smell nice.

Some common poisons found in and around the home:

Medicines
Cleaning products
Batteries
Cigarettes
Plants (indoor
  and outdoor)

Iron pills
Laundry products
Bug and weed killers
Alcohol
Mouthwash

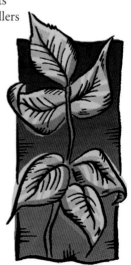

Avoid problems by:

- Keeping children where you can see them at all times, even when you go to answer the telephone. Never leave young children alone, even for just a minute!
- Placing all medicines and household cleaning products out of the reach and sight of children. Keep poisons off of counters.

In case of poisoning:

Take action immediately.

If child has trouble breathing, has seizures, or won't wake up—call 9-1-1 or the local emergency telephone number. Call parent/guardian(s) in all cases.

If ...	Then...
a poison is splashed on the skin or in the **eye(s)**	rinse skin/eye(s) with warm running water for 20 minutes. Take off any splashed clothing. Call the Poison Control Center at 1-800-222-1222.
a poison is **breathed in**	get into fresh air, open doors or windows. Call the Poison Control Center at 1-800-222-1222.
cleaning product or substance causes burning sensation or is swallowed	call the Poison Control Center at 1-800-222-1222. Under the PCC advice, you may give 1 glass of water or milk to drink (unless child is unresponsive, has convulsions, or unable to swallow). Call 9-1-1.
anything else is swallowed	call the Poison Control Center at 1-800-222-1222. Keep the child on his/ her left side to delay the movement of the poison into the small intestine where it can damage the body faster. Keep the child from eating or drinking before calling the Poison Control Center.

Seizures/Convulsions

If a child is prone to seizures, ask the parent/guardian for guidance about what to do and who to call before leaving the child in your care.

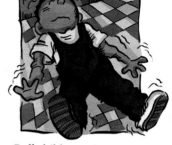

Causes of seizures, other than a seizure disorder (epilepsy), include: high fever, head injury, serious illness, and poisoning.

1. Allow the seizure to occur.
2. Do what you can to prevent injury. Roll child onto left side to allow saliva to drain and keep the tongue from blocking the airway. Cushion child's head with something soft, like a towel.
3. Nothing should be forced between the child's teeth. Allow the child to move freely. The child should not eat or drink until fully alert.
4. After seizure stops, keep victim on his or her side to rest. Recovery is slow and the child will sleep or be drowsy for a while. Most seizures are NOT emergencies and will not require medical help.
5. Always notify the parent(s) or legal guardian(s) when a seizure occurs.
6. Call 9-1-1 when:
   a. Seizures last more than five minutes or if a second seizure occurs.
   b. You have not been told that the child is subject to seizures.
   c. This is a first time seizure (no past seizures).
   d. Any signs of injury or sickness are seen.

Tooth Knocked Out

A child's teeth begin to appear at about six months of age. By age 2½ all teeth will have appeared. These are "baby" teeth. Permanent teeth replace the first set of teeth beginning at about age six and continue until about age 17.

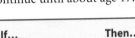

If...	Then...
a tooth has been knocked out	position the child so blood does not compromise the airway. Stop the bleeding with sterile gauze and direct pressure. Pick up the tooth by the crown (the chewing part), not the root. Clean tooth with water. Be gentle. Avoid: a. Soap or chemicals b. Scrubbing the tooth c. Drying the tooth d. Wrapping it in a tissue or cloth Gently place the tooth back in the socket. If the child is able to assist, ask him or her to hold the tooth in place with a finger or tissue. Do not attempt to reinsert a primary/baby tooth. If the child is too young to hold the tooth in place, upset, or if reinserting the tooth is not possible, place the tooth in a glass of milk. Call parent/guardian(s) immediately. It is best for the child to be seen by a dentist within the first 30 minutes after the tooth has been knocked out.

Vomiting

Vomiting is common in children and may be caused by several things. It usually is not serious and quickly passes. Occasional vomiting is not a cause for worry.

1. Children should not eat or drink for 2 to 3 hours after vomiting.
2. After 2 to 3 hours, give 1 to 2 ounces of cool water every half hour to one hour for four feedings. Offer a wet washcloth to keep the mouth and lips moist. If the child begins vomiting again, allow the stomach to rest for another 30 minutes and then start over.
3. Call the parent/guardian(s) if:

   - the child is an infant under six months of age.
   - the child is unable to keep any fluid in stomach for several hours.
   - the child shows signs of dehydration such as dry lips and mouth, a dry diaper for several hours, or small amounts of deep gold colored urine.
   - the child has severe abdominal pain.
   - vomiting is forceful and projectile.
   - there is blood in the vomit.

Recommended Supplies

The parent/guardian(s) may have a first aid kit in their house. However, you should take a small first aid kit along with your other sitter supplies. You can make your own or buy one. Keep child(ren) away from the kit. Some of the contents can be dangerous. Suggested first aid supplies:

- Elastic wrap (2-inch) for wrapping joint and muscle injuries
- Scissors with rounded tips
- Adhesive tape to hold dressings in place
- Sandwich bags for putting ice in and then applying ice bag on joint and muscle injuries

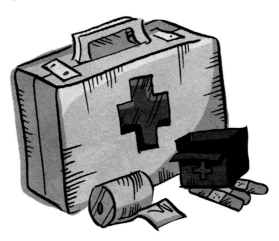

- Dressings (2-inch sterile gauze pads) and adhesive strips of various sizes for covering cuts and scrapes (Children like the ones with designs)
- Antibiotic ointment for burns, cuts, and scrapes
- Hydrocortisone ointment (1%) for rashes that itch
- Tweezers to remove small splinters
- Thermometer (digital or stick on temperature indicators) for measuring fever in children five years and older
- Medical exam gloves (disposable) to protect your hands from blood and reduce chance of infection (2 pairs)
- Face shield or face mask
- Small flashlight
- This manual
- Completed Sitter's Checklist (pages 32, 33) or a list of emergency phone numbers

Kid Fun

Games and Songs

Using these ideas depends upon the child(ren)'s age.

- Draw or color. Bring scrap paper for drawing, and coloring books. Use crayons or washable markers.
- Play a child's audiotape or CD of something fun and lively. Start dancing around the room.
- Children love to play games. The age(s) and number of children determines which you can use.
  - 20 questions
  - Ring Around the Rosy (words are found in the song section)
  - Hide-and-Seek
  - Simon Says
  - Mother May I?
  - I Spy

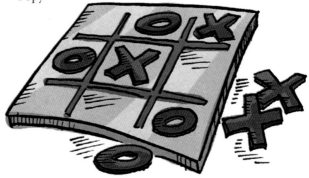

- Play zoo. Have one person pick an animal and act like it while the other(s) guess what animal the person picked.
- Go outside and look at the clouds. Describe them to each other and try to get the other(s) to see which one you're looking at.
- Buy inexpensive books of (1) dot-to-dot, (2) mazes, (3) crossword puzzles, (4) stickers.
- Hangman.
- Tic-Tac-Toe. One player uses Os and another Xs.
- Tag.
- Get child(ren) lined up by a mirror and make faces. See who can make the scariest, silliest, ugliest, and happiest faces.
- Children love when you read to them. Read nursery rhymes from well-known books, such as those of Dr. Seuss and Winnie-the-Pooh. Your local library may have these and many more.
- Children love music. They enjoy singing fun little songs. Here are some words to some all-time favorites:

Bingo

There was a farmer who had a dog
and Bingo was his name
B-I-N-G-O . . . B-I-N-G-O . . . B-I-N-G-O
and Bingo was his name
(spell out B-I-N-G-O)

Head and Shoulders, Knees and Toes

Head and shoulders, knees and toes, knees and toes,
Head and shoulders, knees and toes,
Eyes, ears, mouth, and nose,
Head and shoulders, knees and toes, knees and toes.
(Point to each part of body, repeat song, stop singing a part
   of the body on each repetition but still point to it. Keep
   going until not singing anymore, only pointing.)

If You're Happy and You Know It

If you're happy and you know it clap your hands,
   [clap, clap]
If you're happy and you know it clap your hands,
   [clap, clap]
If you're happy and you know it, and you really want to
   show it,
If you're happy and you know it clap your hands.
   [clap, clap]
If you're happy and you know it stomp your feet…
   [stomp, stomp]

Row, Row, Row Your Boat

Row, row, row your boat
Gently down the stream
Merrily, merrily, merrily, merrily
Life is but a dream.
(This song can be sung as a "round." Group 1 starts the
   song,
Group 2 starts when Group 1 is finished singing the first
   line.
Group 2 will be the last group singing by themselves.)

Ring Around the Rosy

(Children join hands, go around in a circle)
Ring around the rosy
Pocket full of posies
Ashes, ashes
We all fall down!
(Everyone falls down)

Twinkle, Twinkle, Little Star

Twinkle, twinkle, little star,
How I wonder what you are.
Up above the world so high,
Like a diamond in the sky.
Twinkle, twinkle, little star,
How I wonder what you are!

Old MacDonald Had a Farm

Old MacDonald had a farm, E-I-E-I-O
And on this farm he had a cow, E-I-E-I-O.
With a "Moo, Moo" here and a "Moo, Moo" there.
Here a "Moo", there a "Moo," everywhere a "Moo, Moo"
Old MacDonald had a farm, E-I-E-I—O.
Old MacDonald had a farm, E-I-E-I-O
And on his farm he had a _____.

Patty Cake

Patty cake, patty cake baker's man
Bake me a cake as fast as you can.
Roll it and pat it and mark it with a "B"
And put it in the oven for baby and me.

Itsy Bitsy Spider

Itsy bitsy spider went up the water spout.
Down came the rain and washed the spider out.
Out came the sun and it dried up all the rain.
And the Itsy bitsy spider went up the spout again.

Sitter's Busy Bag

This can include items which are fun activities for the
child(ren). Choose things appropriate for the age of the

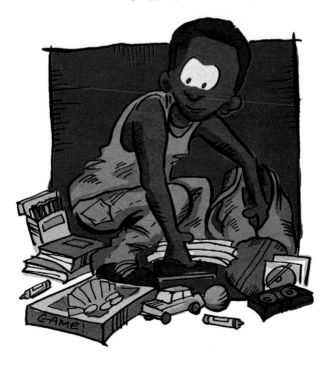

child(ren) you are sitting. Place the items in a container (from a shoebox to a sports bag) to carry them. Suggested Busy Bag items include:

- rubber animals
- plastic or wooden animals with smooth edges
- soft plastic or cloth covered books
- plastic or wooden toy cars or trucks with no small detachable parts
- large rubber ball
- books: nursery rhymes, stories, coloring, dot-to-dot, mazes
- crayons, washable markers
- paper (scrap)
- words to children's songs (see songs in this manual)
- games
- video/DVD/CD

Quick Index